Table of Contents

Preface

We all know "going natural" is a process and definitely takes time and patience. As a matter of fact, many people stop their process once they see how much effort is involved. I am here to help you on *your* natural hair journey. No, it doesn't just happen overnight, although we all wish that it did. With time, patience, and dedication, you will be off to a great start to achieve your natural hair goals in no time.

Allow me to introduce myself. My name is Kayrie, and I am a licensed cosmetologist. I've been in the industry for over 17 years. During that time, I worked in a few shops, had a salon at my home, and styled hair to help pay my way through college. I did a lot of trial and error with my own hair including coloring, perming, relaxing, keratin treatments, and even Brazilian blowouts. You name it, and I have probably tried it. After it all, I realized it's way easier to keep up with your own tresses, not to mention the fact that my hair was a lot healthier by "going natural." Don't get me wrong, I loved my long locks. Still, after repeatedly damaging my tresses with different chemicals, my hair just stopped growing. Has that ever happened to you? Have you found yourself at a standstill with your hair as a result of all the excess manipulation you've put it through over the years? Well, I can tell you something that I discovered in my hair journey.

No matter how much I clipped the ends or spent hundreds of dollars keeping up with treatments, going natural was by far what worked best for me.

If you have made the decision that going natural is best for you too, then you are in the right place. This book is meant to give you the ins and outs of what it takes to not only go natural but grow healthy tresses. If I had a step by step guide to help me on my journey, I would have achieved my goals a lot faster. Nevertheless, I'm here to guide you through the process and give you some tips and tricks that took me years to figure out by myself. Yes, *years.* Why waste years when you can get the full scoop in one book?

I'm not going to overload or overwhelm you with an abundance of information. There's enough info out there to keep you good and busy if that's what you're looking for. I'll keep it sweet, simple, and to the point. This book will give you tons of great information to get you started on your journey.

This book will cover:
- Key points to consider before starting your journey
- A step by step guide on how to achieve your natural hair goals
- How to maintain your natural hair
- Natural hair tips and tricks to help you on your journey
- Natural home remedies and hair cocktails so you can mix up at home

CHAPTER 1
Myth-Busting

There are a few misconceptions about natural hair that I need to clarify before we go any further. There is a lot of "fake news" in the air about going natural, and I'm here to give you some clarification and set the record straight.

Myth: Knowing your hair pattern determines how you care for your hair.

Truthfully, there is some truth to this myth. The keyword is *some*. Sure, knowing your hair pattern is important, and it will be explained more in-depth later on in this book. Whether you have hair pattern 2,3,4, or a combination of a few, the key thing to remember is that *everybody's hair pattern is different*. However, knowing your hair pattern is just part of the battle. There are also other factors to consider when caring for your hair such as *strand size, density, and porosity* to start. That doesn't mean that you don't need to know what your hair pattern is. Knowing your hair pattern is one of the many steps to selecting the best products and regimens to help you on your hair journey. So, find which pattern most resembles your hair, keep that in mind, and let's move forward!

Myth: Going natural will magically make your hair grow longer, thicker, or even prevent hair loss.

The fact that someone said "magically" should be your first red flag. Like the previous myth, there is *some* truth to this statement, however, going natural is not going to automatically solve all of your hair problems. While it won't solve *all* of them, there are several noticeable benefits. Removing chemicals and relaxers will definitely improve the health of your hair. Still, you also have to consider genetics and know key factors to healthy, long, and even thick hair. Be sure to include a consistent regimen that keeps your hair moisturized and nourished. We'll go over that more later.

Myth: Natural hair is easier to keep up with than permed hair.

While natural hair can be easier to "keep up with," it can take more time to develop a regimen and maintain than permed hair. I wouldn't recommend going natural if you don't have the time and patience to commit to maintaining your tresses.

Myth: You don't have to wash kinky, curly, or natural hair.

This myth is absolutely false. It actually makes me chuckle just in writing it. There is no such thing as not needing to wash your hair because of your hair type. What is true is that natural hair doesn't require a harsh cleansing method where oils are stripped from the hair. Nevertheless, ALL hair should be washed regularly. Not washing hair regularly can lead to build-up on your hair and scalp, which can leave your hair feeling and looking dry and dull over time. Not to mention that it won't smell too great.

Myth: Oils moisturize natural hair.

A common misconception that is easy to see why it's misconstrued. What oils can do is seal and lock moisture into your hair, but oils don't actually provide the moisture you *need*. On the contrary, oils actually repel moisture, which is why it keeps the moisture in your hair. Applying oils without moisturizing first can lead to dry, crunchy hair. Trust me, you do not want to deal with excess dryness while you're going natural.

Myth: Protective hair styles are the best way to help you grow or transition your hair.

As much as I love protective styling, this is not the most accurate statement. Don't get me wrong, *protective styles* are a great way to assist you in transitioning and growing your hair out, but they shouldn't be your only resort. Leaving your hair in a protective style for long periods of time can lead to breakage and damage to the hair. You can read more about protective styles in the next chapter of this book.

Now that we got a few myths and misconceptions about natural hair out of the way, let's get started with some hair basics!

CHAPTER 2
The Basics About Natural Hair

Now you may be wondering, what do you mean when you say, "natural hair"? Let me break it down for you. *Natural hair* is hair that has not been "altered." When referring to altered, I mean it has not been processed by any type of chemicals, including *straighteners, relaxers,* and *texturizers.* Some have incorrectly associated pressed hair with processed hair; however, that isn't the case. Pressed hair is considered natural because it returns to its natural state after being washed.

Natural hair can range from straight, wavy, to kinky and curly. It requires frequent conditioning, moisturizing, and applying the least amount of direct heat as possible. There are a lot of different ways to style natural hair; a few popular hairstyles are twists, braids, cornrows, afros, bantu knots, finger coils, and wash and go's.

Ready to go natural? "Going natural" is not as easy as it sounds. There are a few things to consider before starting the journey. You should take ALL of the following factors into consideration when thinking of going natural to determine if you are ready to take that BIG step.

Things to consider when going natural:

The Big Chop – The big chop or BC is when you choose to cut all of your processed hair off and have a "fresh start." This seems like the simplest way to go but not necessarily the easiest. You may prefer to keep your locks and go through a "transition." From there, you gradually cut your hair little by little until all of the chemically processed hair is gone.

Transitioning – Transitioning is the period you go through when trying to get the chemicals out of your hair. This can be done by rocking your transitioning curls or wearing a *protective hairstyle.*

Learning Your Pattern – It is imperative that you get to know your natural hair pattern, so you know the best styles and products that work on your hair.

Cost – Be ready to spend a few dollars on styling products and finding what products work best for your hair. Remember, everyone's hair is different and unique.

Shrinkage – A lot of time when going natural, you have to deal with shrinkage. Some ladies may be okay with it, while others may want to rock a *protective hairstyle.*

Process – Know that going natural is a process, and it doesn't happen overnight. Even if you end up doing a big chop, you still have to take the time to learn your hair and what styles or products work best for you. It takes time and patience to get it just right!

Wash Day – Wash day is also a process. You must be willing and able to learn your process and develop a daily or weekly routine.

CHAPTER 3
Different Hair Types and Patterns

There are four different hair types: **straight, wavy, curly, kinky**. It is important to know your hair type so you can determine how to care for it. Knowing your hair texture dictates how often you wash your hair, what products to use, and what styles work best for you.

How do I know what type of hair type I have?

Every hair texture is different, and hair texture is determined by your curl pattern. A curl pattern is the shape of the curl as it naturally grows from the scalp. The shape or pattern is determined by your hair follicle.

How to determine curl pattern:

To determine your natural curl pattern, start with wet hair.
Wavy hair appears straight when wet and will shrink 10% when dry.
Curly hair is wavy when wet and will shrink 25% when dry.
Coily hair has tight coils when wet with major shrinkage up to 50% when dry.

The next thing you need to understand is how these curl patterns coincide with the hair types, which are represented by numbers.

Type 1 is straight hair. There is no wave whatsoever.
Tips: Proper shampooing is important to maintaining healthy, straight hair. Use a mild shampoo and avoid brushing wet hair. Brushing may cause hair to stretch and break. Try using fingers

or a wide-tooth comb to remove knots instead. Straight hair is prone to split ends, so getting ends trimmed every 4 to 6 weeks is best.

Type 2 is wavy hair and has a slight bump and a visible S pattern.

Tips: Use lightweight products to boost hydration and hold waves. Natural oils are great for your hair and scalp, but they can also make the hair look greasy. Try using pre-poo treatments and washing out after. Additionally, deep condition hair at least every 2 weeks.

Types of Waves: 2A, 2B, 2C
2A is easily manipulated to be straight because the wave is so loose. 2B has a slightly more noticeable wave and a consistent S-shape. 2C has S-shapes that are very apparent; large waves can appear as ringlets.

Best Styling Products: mousse, foam, lightweight gels and creams, and serums.

Type 3 is curly hair with a spiral shape; curls range from loose to tight.

Tips: Wash your hair no more than twice a week and deep condition every 4th or 5th wash. If your hair gets greasy mid-week, use a co-wash in between washes and light oils to seal in moisture.

Types of Curls: 3A, 3B, 3C
3A is wavy when wet and springs into curls when dry. 3B curls are the size of a sharpie and tighter than 3A ringlets. Curls of this type dry quickly. 3C are corkscrew curls the size of pencils. Try to use more cream than gel because gel tends to dry this type of hair out, whereas cream gives more moisture. Feel free to refresh with conditioner and/or water as needed.

Styling products: curling creams, "curl enhancing" mousse, light to medium weight gels, and curl milks.

Type 4 is coily hair which is the tightest among all hair types;

curls spring straight from the scalp.

Tips: Keep curls moisturized and opt for methods that stretch curls. Avoid heavy products so hair can remain bouncy. Coily hair dries out quickly, so be sure to keep curls moisturized. Use a lot of conditioner on wet hair to help with moisture and detangling. Moisturize daily with a leave-in conditioner, moisturizer, or steam. Deep condition every 1-2 weeks and opt for methods that stretch curls.

Styling products: Shampoos and products that provide a lot of moisture, protection, and deep conditioning. Look for hydrating ingredients that will seal the hair such as products that contain humectants, glycerin, honey and butters. Avoid heavy waxes, parabens, sodium chloride, alcohols and anything that dries or coats the hair.

CHAPTER 4
Good vs. Bad ingredients in Hair Products

Knowing what's in your hair products is imperative. With so many different products on the market, you may be wondering which one should you choose? Which ingredients are good for your hair? What ingredients should you avoid? I'm about to share all those answers below.

Ingredients to avoid in hair products

Here are a few ingredients that you should try to avoid when choosing your hair products and why.

Parabens - Parabens are man-made chemicals created to preserve the formula of different hair products so they will last longer. They are of a sufficiently high molecular weight to prevent evaporation. In other words, it's a filler to extend the shelf life of a product. Parabens can lead to water loss from the hair, which can cause frizz and dryness.

Alcohols - Isopropyl alcohol and other alcohols have been known to cause excessive dryness to the hair. This alcohol is found in household cleaners, including antifreeze. Additionally, this hair product ingredient can also dissolve oils, which is a necessity for natural hair to flourish.

Formaldehyde & Formaldehyde Releasers - Formaldehydes are preservatives placed into your cosmetics and hair products meant to prevent the growth of bacteria. A formaldehyde-releaser will typically be one of the last ingredients on the label. The reason you don't want these in your hair is because these chemicals can be absorbed through the skin and have been linked to cancer and allergic skin reactions.

Sulfates - Sulfates are a salt formed from sulfuric acid. They are typically found in shampoos and are used to completely remove the hair of build-up and other elements. Sulfates are meant to cleanse the hair entirely of everything, including the oils your hair naturally produces. Sulfates stripping the hair of their natural oils can lead to more dryness and duller-looking hair.

Silicones - Be aware of any ingredients that end in "-cone" on your natural hair products. Silicones, like sulfates, aren't entirely terrible for your hair. Still, what they *can* do is cause build-up over time, creating dull, brittle natural hair.

Mineral Oil - Mineral oil is an oil produced from petroleum. It is used for many things in the cosmetics industry. Because of its blocking and clogging effect on the hair follicles, this oil can cause more build-up than anything else.

Synthetic Fragrance / Perfumes - A lot of the times, these synthetic scents that smell fruity or flowery are formulated with chemicals and preservatives to get that aroma. While they may smell nice, these scents can cause allergic irritations and breakouts on the skin. If you wish to find a product that contains a smell-good scent, try products that are "naturally" scented with essential oils and/or natural extracts.

Polyethylene Glycol (PGE) & Propylene Glycol (PG) - Polyethylene Glycol & Propylene Glycol are water-soluble compounds found in hair products. PG is found in some foods, and antifreeze can also contain this ingredient. Both compounds have been found to make it easier for other ingredients to penetrate the skin and be absorbed into the bloodstream when used in higher concentrations. I think it's safe to assume that there are certain ingredients you absolutely do not want to enter your body, which is why you need to steer clear of PG and PGE.

Good ingredients

Now that you've seen the bad ingredients, let me introduce you to some of the better ones. The following ingredients are good for your hair, so look for these when choosing your hair products.

Water - Make sure it's listed as one of the first few ingredients. To provide moisture to your tresses, there needs to be water present. Whether to provide, absorb, or retain that moisture, water has to be the main ingredient. Specifically, water should be listed as the first ingredient or at least towards the very top, showing that it is most prevalent. Water being listed as an ingredient ensures that your strands are going to receive as much moisture as possible.

Coconut Oil, Avocado Oil, Olive Oil - All of these oils are moisturizing oils. Most natural oils for hair serve as sealants, meaning they help to seal in moisture and provide moisturizing properties. They are able to penetrate the hair shaft with the help of water. These are good ingredients to look for in your natural hair products that will help your hair retain softness, shine, and moisture.

Glycerin / Vegetable Glycerin - You have probably seen glycerin on the label of a few of your favorite hair products. It is another one of the good ingredients to look for in natural hair products because they are humectants, meaning they draw in moisture. Glycerin and vegetable glycerin are essentially the same thing. The only difference is that one comes from an animal.

Honey- Honey is another healthy choice to add to the list of good ingredients. When used on natural hair, it leaves your hair feeling smooth, just like regular honey. Honey is a natural humectant, helping to absorb and retain moisture. There are nourishing benefits, including antibacterial properties which help to alleviate certain scalp conditions

Shea Butter - Shea butter is a common yet useful ingredient to look for in your natural hair products. It is rich in vitamins and minerals, including omega fatty acids that give it its moisturizing properties. These nutrients help the product to penetrate the hair shaft, serving as both a moisturizer and a sealant.

Natural Extracts - You may notice multiple ingredients ending in "extract" on your hair product labels. Natural extracts are additional ingredients to look for in natural hair products. The majority of these extracts are derivatives from natural sources, including plants, seeds, fruits, and more. It will typically list in parentheses the source it is extracted from. The benefits of these natural extracts include shine, anti-aging properties, reduced shedding, and other things your hair craves. If you see natural extracts on the label, that's a good indication that your hair will love it.

Biotin - Our hair strands are comprised of a protein called keratin. Keratin helps to keep your hair strands healthy and in-tact. The amino acids derived from biotin aid in the composition of keratin, contributing to hair health and growth.

Castor Seed Oil - Not only is this vegetable oil a humectant, but castor oil also has antifungal properties. This will ensure a clean scalp, with the hair follicles clear and prepared for better hair growth.

Avocado/Avocado Oil - Many natural hair products use avocado since it's packed with vitamins A, D, and E. Avocado also contains more potassium than bananas. Easily absorbed into the skin, avocado oil is a quick way to get multiple nutrients onto your scalp for improved hair growth.

There you have all the good and bad ingredients that you need to be aware of as you go on your natural hair journey. Next, we're going to talk about how you should approach wash days.

CHAPTER 5

Shampoo and Pre-poo

Natural hair terms can be confusing at times. Especially when you have so many gurus trying to tell you what's what. Trust me, I get it. I was there once too. No need to try to make sense out of the different terms floating around. I'm here to break each one down to you.

First and foremost, let's start with shampoo. Whether you're processed or natural, if you are cleansing your hair, you're familiar with regular shampoo. But, do you know just how important it is as it pertains to natural hair? Let's look at the definition below.

Shampoo – Shampoo is a hair care cleansing product, in a liquid form, used for cleaning hair. Apply shampoo to wet hair, massage through hair and scalp, and rinse out. When picking shampoo, you want to be sure to pick one that does not strip your hair of all of its moisture. Commercial, medicated, and dandruff shampoos tend to be filled with cleansing agents that strip your hair, leaving it dry after shampooing. Remember the ingredients we talked about to avoid? You'll need to use the knowledge here.

You should try to use a mild shampoo to help preserve the health of your hair. A mild shampoo means a shampoo that doesn't contain harmful chemicals and will not damage hair, even if it is used every day. Mild shampoos have a naturally beneficial effect on our hair and should not cause any irritation to the skin or scalp. If you shampoo your hair and it has a "squeaky clean" feeling afterward, it's likely that you stripped your hair of a lot of natural oils. Don't stress too much; you can still fix it. A deep conditioning treatment is definitely recommended to restore the moisture. Deep conditioning will be discussed more in-depth in chapter 6.

How to use shampoo:

Clarifying Shampoo – Clarifying shampoos are like a reset button for your hair. Unlike regular shampoos, clarifying shampoos are designed to remove surface-level gunk and grime, rather than condition and smooth. Clarifying shampoos deep cleanse your hair from chemicals, waxes, and residue left behind by your hair products, which means that they provide a much deeper clean. This type of shampoo is not for everyday use and can be used once no more than twice a month. Be sure to balance out with a deep conditioner.

How to use clarifying shampoo
1) Wet hair
2) Focus on roots, where most of the build-up tends to be worse.
3) Massage shampoo into the scalp, working your way down to the ends.
4) Follow up with a conditioner, deep conditioner, or even a mask to help restore moisture.

Pre-Poo – Pre-poo is the process of applying treatment to the hair before the shampooing. The purpose of this treatment is to provide your hair with a protective layer. This can be helpful because depending on which shampoo you use, moisture can be stripped from the hair.

Pre-poo tends to be popular with curly or kinky hair, but in actuality, any hair type can benefit from a pre-poo treatment. Benefits of pre-pooing include adding extra moisture to dry hair, promoting softer, vibrant hair, easier to detangle, and boosting the effects of the conditioner, resulting in stronger hair and less breakage. The pre-poos process is fairly simple; just follow the steps below.

How to pre-poo

1.) Start off by dividing your hair into four to eight sections, depending on the length and thickness. Sections will make it easier to distribute product evenly throughout your hair.
2.) Coat your hair with the product from root to ends. After applying product, detangle each section of hair with a wide-tooth comb, starting with the roots first and working your way up to the scalp.
3.) Leave treatment in hair for a least 30 minutes before shampooing. Keep in mind that the longer you pre-poo, the better. You can pre-poo earlier in the day and shampoo several hours later, or you can even leave the treatment in overnight. If you do choose to leave it in overnight, be sure to wear some type of protective gear on your hair such as a scarf or a bonnet and wash your hair in the morning.
4.) Once you wash your hair, be sure to wash your hair thoroughly. Get all the product out to prevent residue.

Types of pre-poo treatments

There are several pre-poo treatments out there for you to choose from. Take a look below at some of the most common.

Pre-poo oils - These are good if you want to add moisture to straight or curly hair. Oils help repair damage caused by heat, chemicals, or coloring. Much of these oils will remain on your hair after washing since oils don't easily rinse away after shampooing. Examples of pre-poo oils include avocado, coconut, almond, and argan oils.

Pre-poo aloe vera gels - Aloe vera gel is also another option to increase moisture in the hair. Aloe vera is good if you are having problems with dandruff. Aloe vera gel can reduce inflammation and itchiness caused by dandruff and contains antifungal properties.

Pre-Poo Butters - Pre-poo butters include shea butter, cocoa butter, mango butter, and hempseed butter. Each one helps strengthen the hair shaft and prevents breakage caused by chemical, heat, or color treatments. They can also help rebuild hair follicles, promoting hair growth and fullness. Not only do they strengthen hair, but they also provide moisture for shinier and softer hair.

CHAPTER 8
Masks and Treatments - The Purpose and Benefits

What is a mask?

A hair mask is a deep conditioning treatment that helps heal damaged hair. Hair masks are for all types of hair. Depending on what you're looking for, the choices are endless. Whether purchasing or making your own hair mask, you should look for ingredients such as jojoba oil and almond oil, which add moisture to your hair. There are food products you can use at home to make your own masks such as avocados, bananas, and honey, which help restore nutrients to hair. Yogurt is good for treating dull and damaged hair and prevent dandruff, while egg yolks provide moisture. We have several DIY recipes in chapter 15 of this book if you want to try it at home.

How often you apply a hair mask is determined by how damaged your hair is and what your hair routine looks like. For most hair types, once a week should suffice just fine, but if you are applying heat to your hair daily, you may want to use them more often or even a more intense method. Be careful not to overuse masks; it can leave you with oily, limp, or dull hair if done too often. Hair masks are easy to add to your normal hair routine, and they normally take the place of your conditioner.

How to use a hair mask:
1) Shampoo and rinse your hair.
2) Apply a generous amount of the mask to your hair.
3) Wait 3-5 minutes or the allotted amount of time as directed on the product label.

4) Rinse.

5) Towel dry and style hair as usual.

What is a hair treatment?

A hair treatment is not to be confused with a conditioner. A hair treatment penetrates the hair, restoring and maintaining internal strength. There are 2 types of treatments: reconstructors and moisturizers.

Reconstructors make the hair stronger and are generally protein-based. These are good for chemically damaged, breaking, or weak hair types.

Moisturizers are the most common type of treatments. They balance the moisture content of the cortex (middle) of your hair. These are good for frizzy and dry hair, or if you have curly hair and lack bounce.

Tips for using hair treatments:

-   Be sure to read label before using it on your hair. Don't assume you know what you are doing.
-   Treatments should be used according to the instructions on the label.
-   Use the hair treatment designed to reach whichever hair goal you are trying to achieve, whether it's for hydration, strength, definition, or hair growth.

CHAPTER 6

Co-Washing and Scrubs

Co-washing. What is it anyway? To be blunt, co-washing is washing your hair solely with conditioner. If you have an afro, curly, kinky, mixed textured, or extremely dry hair, you may benefit from co-washing. Like I stated earlier, harsh shampoos like those containing sulfates have the tendency to strip the hair of its natural oils, leaving your hair dry and more prone to breakage. By substituting some of your shampoo regimens with co-washing, you can maintain moisture and overall healthy hair. Let's be clear: co-washing isn't the same as skipping shampooing and just using conditioner all the time. Co-washing is using conditioner in the place of shampoo. When choosing a co-wash, be sure to pick one that doesn't contain silicone. Silicone can add shine but, over time, leaves build-up. Build-up causes your hair to feel heavy and dull.

How to co-wash hair:
    1) Wet hair.
    2) Take about a teaspoon amount of conditioner and massage through the scalp, like you would shampoo.
    3) Take a regular amount of conditioner and condition hair as usual. Be sure to use a wide-tooth comb to detangle hair.
    4) You can rinse the conditioner out entirely, or you can also rinse for a few seconds and leave hair still slightly coated.

Over time, if you notice any product build-up, be sure to cleanse hair with a clarifying shampoo.

Scrubs. What are they, and why and how should I use them?

Scalp scrubs are great for your hair. Similar to facial and body scrubs, they exfoliate dead skin cells on your scalp. Scrubs will get rid of product build-up and fight off excess oil, leaving your hair healthy, thick, and shiny. Keep in mind that scalp scrubs aren't for everyone, and not everyone benefits from using them. Scalp scrubs aren't good if you suffer from skin conditions on the scalp such as psoriasis, acne, eczema, or have any cuts or sores. If you don't have any skin irritations, here's a good way to tell if you need a scalp scrub or not.

You may want to consider a scrub if:
- You don't wash all the product out of your hair.
- You use dry shampoo.
- You have oil, sweat, or build-up on your scalp.
- You have finer hair and are more prone to build-up.

How to use scalp scrub:
1) Wet hair and section.
2) Apply generous amount to scalp.
3) Scrub scalp with fingertips. Use fingertips, brush, or glove to help exfoliate.
4) Rub in a gentle circular motion.
5) Rinse thoroughly, then follow-up with shampoo and conditioner. Use more than once a week or every other week for best results.

CHAPTER 7

Detangling and Deep Conditioning

Detangling

Detangling is the act of removing tangles from the hair. It can be one of the most important steps to help keep your hair healthy and strong.

When dealing with naturally curly, kinky hair, there are a few things to keep in mind.

- *Start from the ends and work your way up to the roots.* You always want to start at the ends of your hair and work your way up to the roots to prevent damage.
- *Detangling in the shower is ideal.* It's always a good idea to detangle while your hair is wet, and detangling in the shower doesn't hurt. Apply conditioner to your hair and use a wide-tooth comb, starting from the ends and working your way up to the roots.
- *Detangle before you shampoo.* If your curls get tangled easily, detangle before your shampoo, then shampoo and condition.
- After detangling your hair, use a moisturizer to prevent your hair from drying out.

Deep Conditioning

So, you may be wondering, what is the purpose of deep conditioning, and why do you need to do it?

There are several benefits to deep conditioning daily. First off, it is important to know that deep conditioning is important for *all* hair types. Deep conditioning keeps the hair moisturized, builds up strength, prevents damage from heat and styling tools, and helps replace moisture and vital proteins in the hair shaft. Deep conditioning also assists with restoring luster, shine, and strength to your hair. Whether your hair is bone straight or coily, you need to be deep conditioning on a regular.

There are two different types of deep conditioning: moisture and protein. Both are very beneficial and serve specific purposes. *Moisturizing* deep conditioners contain humectants that attract water and are absorbed into the hair. *Protein* deep conditioners are considered heavy hitters because they are used to help increase the diameter of the hair with a coating action. Protein deep conditioners can also be called treatments as they contain proteins to help strengthen the hair. Protein hardens the cuticle layer of your hair and also puts a protective barrier around each strand. Protein deep conditioners help increase elasticity and improve the overall appearance of your hair.

Tips: Use protein deep conditioner if hair is color-treated, damaged, or showing signs of weakness. Use a protein deep conditioner once a month or every 2 months depending upon the condition of your hair.

How to Apply Deep Conditioner:

-   Start with clean wet hair.
-   Apply deep conditioner to hair in sections, starting with the ends and working your way up to the roots.
-   Leave conditioner in for 15-30 minutes (or longer depending on directions). Use heat for the best results
-   Rinse with cool water.

5 Reasons Why Deep Conditioning is Important

There are several reasons why deep conditioning is important. Here are a few below:

Prevents Damage - Deep conditioning helps to reduce breakage and split ends, improves your hair's health, and helps maintain healthy hair overall.

Promotes Elasticity - Deep conditioning helps prevent breakage and allows you to improve the elasticity of your hair.

Restores Natural Shine - Deep conditioning penetrates the hair shaft and helps to restore the natural shine to the hair.

Adds Moisture - Deep conditioning adds moisture, and moisture is the key to healthy hair. If your hair is not properly moisturized, it may become dry and brittle, making it prone to breakage. Deep conditioning helps keep your curls strong and ensures your hair retains the moisture it needs to stay healthy.

Helps Color-Treated Hair - Color can be detrimental to your hair, and it can also alter your hair strand's structure. When this happens, your hair becomes weak and leaves it open to dryness and breakage. Help avoid damage by deep conditioning your hair regularly.

The Do's and Don'ts of Deep Conditioning

Do's:
- *Deep condition on a regular basis.*
  - Suggested Use: If you're a "pro," deep condition every other week. If you're transitioning, deep condition once or twice a week.
- *Apply heat to help speed up the process.* Using at least 35 degrees Celsius increases amount of effectiveness and absorption.
- *Try heating up the conditioner.* This assists in its effectiveness when used.
- *Alternate between protein and moisturizing deep conditioning treatments.* You need both to maintain optimum hair health.
- *Add steam.* Adding steam heats up the cuticle, allowing better penetration of conditioner.
- *Rinse with cool or cold water.* This will close the hair cuticle and

keep the moisture in your hair.
- *Read the ingredients.* It's always important to know what you are putting on your hair.
- *Focus on your ends first.* Allow them time to soak up the ingredients.
- *When applying conditioner, blot off the excess water in your hair.* The conditioner will slide off if your hair is too wet, and it won't penetrate well.

Don't:
- *Overdo it.* No need to deep condition overnight or for hours; 15 minutes minimum or one hour max unless otherwise stated.
- *Multitask.* Don't use a co-wash or leave-in conditioner as a deep conditioner. They are two different steps in the process, so perform each one separately.
- *Forget to wash it out.* Leaving conditioner on your hair can lead to build-up.
- *Go outside of your budget.* It can get pricey trying to find the right products for your hair. Be wise with your spending.
- *Invite bacteria.* Homemade remedies are good for a week max if refrigerated. Try to mix enough for one single-use to prevent bacteria in your concoctions.
- *Be fooled.* Only the first 5 ingredients have the greatest impact on your hair. Everything else is fluff.

CHAPTER 9
Moisturizers

The purpose of using a moisturizer is just that, to add moisture to your hair. *Leave in moisturizers are designed to add moisture to your hair.*

There are several factors that can cause dry hair:
- The scalp doesn't produce enough natural oil to keep hair moisturized.
- The condition or structure of your hair is causing the moisture to escape.
- Too many chemicals can cause dry hair such as perms, relaxers, highlights, and color.
- Thermal abuse can lead to dry hair. This includes the use of flat irons, curling irons, and blow dryers. High temperatures can and will strip strands of their natural moisture. You don't want this to happen to you.
  - Tips to prevent thermal abuse:
    - *Use a protective formula before applying heat to your hair.* These products provide a barrier between heat and thermal tools and can help prevent dry hair.
    - *Consider using ionic thermal tools.* It's important to understand that positive and negative ions exist. When the hair is wet, hair is positively charged. Ionic hair tools inject the hair with negative ions, allowing water molecules to penetrate deep into the hair. This results in rehydrated hair.

- *Turn down the heat.* Quality hair tools normally feature temperature settings. If your hair is dry, use a lower setting. By using a lower setting now, your hair will thank you later.
- *Take a break from heat altogether.* Consider trying a protective hairstyle such as buns, braids, or bantu knots that don't require heat.

Exposing your hair to too much sun, salt water, chlorine, dry air, and wind can cause dryness as well.

- Tips for preventing dryness:
  - *Apply UV protection to your hair.* Look for products or sprays that offer UV protection.
  - *Waterproof your dry hair.* Try coating your hair with a thick conditioning or treatment oil and cover it with a swim cap before jumping into the beach or pool.
  - *Wear a cute hat or scarf over your hair.* Help protect your hair from the sun and UV rays that can cause color to fade and hair to dry.
  - *Set up your conditioning routine.* This is always recommended but especially with harsh weather. Conditioning weekly is always a good start.

Bad brushes can cause dry hair and poorly made brushes that have uneven, jagged bristles can cause hair to tear, leading to moisture loss.

- Tips for brushes:
  - *Never brush hair when it's wet.* Hair is most vulnerable when it is wet and can be broken easily by the bristles on a brush.
  - *Use a wide-tooth comb instead.* Using a wide tooth comb is best for curls because it re-

duces breakage. Start with the ends and working your way up to the roots when detangling.

Moisturizing Tips for Different Hair Types

Curly hair tends to be dryer than other types of hair because of its structure. Due to the shape of the curls, it takes longer for the oil from the scalp to make its way through the length of the hair. Curly hair needs moistures the most!

Tips for Dry Curly Hair:
- *Prime before styling.* If you use a styling or blowout cream before styling, try using a leave-in moisturizing formula as well for double penetration and an extra shot of moisture.
- *Spritz then seal your hair with water then conditioner.* Try filling a water bottle with two-thirds water and one-third moisturizing spray-on conditioner. Mist your hair until damp, then seal in moisture with rich conditioning cream or oil.
- *Take the time out for a weekly hot oil treatment.* Apply an oil formula treatment to your dry hair and comb through with a wide-tooth comb. Cover your hair with a plastic cap and sit under a dryer, in a warm room, or in the sun for 20-30 minutes. Afterward, rinse, shampoo, and condition.

Similar to curly hair, the structure of *coarse, thick hair* often leads to dryness. The volume and shape make it hard for this hair type to be moisturized by scalps natural oils.

Tips for Moisturizing Thick Coarse Dry Hair
- *Use pre-styling creams and treatment oils before using thermal tools.* Apply rich styling formulas or oils to your damp hair before blow-drying or applying heat. Use a lower temperature setting in your blow dryer.
- *Layer your conditioners.* Use a rich rinse-out conditioner after every shampoo and follow up with a moisturizing leave-in spray before styling.
- *Take your vitamins.* Try adding hair vitamins to your diet that

contain Vitamin B, folic acid, biotin, magnesium, sulfur, and zinc.

Fine hair can become dry; be careful when moisturizing not to weigh hair down.

Tips for Moisturizing Fine Dry Hair
- *Choose a conditioner for fine hair.* This should be a lightweight and rinseable conditioner, so it doesn't weigh hair down or cause it to flatten.
- *Avoid the roots.* Fine hair tends to be dry on the ends, so try to apply conditioner to dry areas and skip the roots to avoid weighing down the hair or causing it to become oily.

CHAPTER 10

Oils: Moisturizing and Sealants

The purpose of an oil sealant is to provide moisture and reduce breakage. When thick or heavy oils are applied to hair, it creates a seal. A seal is a barrier that helps prevent moisture from getting out. Keep in mind that it can also prevent moisture from coming in. There are two types of oils: moisturizing and sealant oils.

Moisturizing oils are able to penetrate the hair shaft. These oils work best when used with a water-based leave-in conditioner or with water by itself. The oils are great for hot oil treatments and pre-poo treatments because they don't leave a film on your hair; they actually penetrate the hair.

Examples of moisturizing oils are as follows:

- *Coconut Oil* – This is a common oil used in many natural beauty products. It's naturally antibacterial and antifungal, great for skin, and an excellent moisturizer. On top of that, it can penetrate the shaft better than other oils. It's most effective when used with water or water-based leave-ins.

- *Olive Oil* – This oil can have a major moisturizing effect. It makes tresses soft and strengthens each strand by penetrating the hair shaft and retaining moisture. It also leaves your hair shiny because it helps smooth the outer cuticle layer of your hair.

- *Avocado Oil* - This oil is ideal for dry hair that is caused by heat or environmental factors. It strengthens hair because of its high vitamin E content and prevents breakage. Avocado oil is lighter than olive oil and will absorb into the cuticle without weighing your hair down. It's good to use as a pre-poo treatment.

Sealant oils are unable to penetrate the hair shaft. They work best when applied after a good moisturizer and are used to seal in the moisture already applied. The seal created helps moisture from getting out. It's best to use sealing oils after the hair is already moisturized to make sure that any moisture you put in your hair stays locked in.

Example of sealant oils are:
- *Jamaican Black Castor Oil (JBCO)* – This is one of the best sealant oils you can use with natural hair. JBCO helps soften hairs while drawing out toxins and impurities that prevent hair growth. This oil is thick and a great sealant for thicker texture hair.
- *Jojoba Oil* – This is a fairly light oil that is most effective in sealing moisture added during wash day. Jojoba is good for people with dry or flaky scalps to help restore proper pH to your hair.
- *Grapeseed Oil* – This is an extremely light oil and has the ability to withstand high amounts of heat. This oil is best for women with finer or thinner strands who want to seal in moisture without weighing down hair or leaving it oily or greasy.

Here is a quick guide to using oils:
- **Moisturizing/penetrating oils**: Coconut oil, Sunflower oil, and Palm Kernel oil
- **Partially penetrating and sealing oils**: Avocado oil, Olive oil, and Argan oil

- **Sealing oils**: Jojoba oil, Jamaican Black Castor oil, Grapeseed oil

CHAPTER 11
Curly Hair Products: Curl Smoothies, Pomades, Hair Milk, Mousses, Curl Activators

Curl Smoothies
The primary function is to soften, moisturize, refresh, detangle, condition, and style hair. Different brands use smoothies in various ways, including conditioners, styles, and refreshers. Reading the ingredient list is a great way to see if the smoothie is a good match for your strands.

Pomades
Pomades are in the same class of stylers as gel and curl definers. Pomades are good for hold, shine, and controlling frizz. Also, you will see many use pomades for more polished styles or updos. Pomades lock in moisture and often have wax in them to help with hold.

Hair Milk
Hair milk is in the same category as hair lotion, milkshakes, and a leave-in conditioner. These products are light and are meant to refresh. They can be used daily to add moisture. Hair milk has a goal of being a hydrating leave-in that aids in detangling and combating frizz. Hair milk tends to have a milk-like consistency (hence the name) and rejuvenates your thirsty strands. Different brands will incorporate vitamins, oils, and herbs to help bring your curls back to life.

Curl Activators
Curl activators not only provide moisture to fight frizz and promote shine, but they also really help define your curls. As the

name implies, curl activators are essential for springy and tight curls, but other types of curls and waves can benefit from it too.

There are a few considerations you should take into account if you want to use curl activators. When choosing your curl activator, you should definitely know your hair type. There are several different formulas, such as cream, custards, sprays. Each formula has a different consistency, and the three main types are outlined below:
- *Cream* is the most common form of an activator. Creams are usually a thick consistency and offer plenty of moisture.
- *Custards* are a cross between gels and creams. They have a lighter consistency than creams but don't dry the hair out like gel.
- *Sprays* have a liquid consistency and are often used as a primer for other hair products. They don't leave behind a greasy or sticky residue.

Mousses
Mousses aren't heavy on the hair and are great for reviving curl definition and fighting frizz. Mousses are good for fine hair because they don't weigh hair down and work best when applied to wet hair. It can also be used under gel on wet hair for looser patterns.

CHAPTER 12
Hair Gel vs. Curl Creams

Curl Creams

Curls Creams are designed to moisturize, smooth, and define your curls. Curl creams aid in providing soft hold and definition to your curls. They are designed to allow your hair to be moisturized from the inside out and won't leave you with flakes or frizz. They can be more nourishing than gels and leave less build-up than other products. They may not provide as much hold as gels, so you may want to consider using a little of both if you want your curls to last.

It is recommended to apply creams to soaking wet hair for maximum curl definition. Applying your curl cream is similar to applying your gel.

How to use curl creams:
1) After washing your hair, section it off into 3-5 sections.
2) While hair is wet, apply a generous amount of product to each section of hair.
3) Work the cream from the root to the ends of your hair.
4) Air dry your hair or use a diffuser.

Hair Gels

Hair Gels have the main function of holding and setting the hair. Even though all gels have the same purpose, they are not created equal. The use of gel is optional. The gel you choose will depend on the styling needs of your tresses. For a light hold, try using a watery gel or one with a loose consistency. For a stronger hold or for keeping edges "laid" or held smooth without reverting back to curls, choose a gel with a thicker consistency. Gels can also be used to define your curl pattern and make your curls "pop." Check the label of the gel to see what type of hold it provides. Please keep in mind that gel is the final styling product and should be applied to your hair when it is wet.

How to apply gel to curly or wavy hair for styling (Method 1):

1) Use curl cream or whatever products you normally use in your routine to style your hair.
2) Use a cotton t-shirt or microfiber hair towel to scrunch curls up and remove excess water.
3) Apply a quarter-size amount of gel to the palm of your hands, rub them together, and apply to the ends of your hair by scrunching in a upward motion.
4) Use the palm of your hands to smooth down gel and distribute evenly through hair.
5) Air dry or diffuse hair. Once hair is completely dry, "scrunch out the crunch."

How to apply gel to curly or wavy hair for styling

(Method 2):

1) Use curl cream or whatever products you normally use in your routine to style your hair.
2) Use gel as the last layer of product to apply to your hair when styling.
3) After hair is set, spray with a water bottle to re-dampen (not soaking wet). Apply 1-2 quarter amounts of gel to the palm of your hands.
4) Apply gel to hair using an upward scrunching motion.
5) Use a cotton t-shirt or microfiber towel to scrunch excess water and product out of your hair.
6) Air dry or diffuse hair. Once hair is completely dry, "scrunch out the crunch."

CHAPTER 13
The Process: Finding out which process works best for you

There are a few different options when styling your hair while wet. It's just a matter of finding out which option works best for you. Just because it works for one person does not mean it will work for you and vice versa. Figuring out the right curly hair routine is the hardest part, especially because everyone's hair is different.

Wash and Go Method
This method is probably the simplest method of them all. It's also the easiest if you're pressed for time.

How to style your hair with the wash and go method:
1) Wet or wash and condition your hair.
2) Apply product to your hair while wet. Be sure to use your leave-in conditioner and your favorite styling product.
3) Scrunch your hair to encourage curl pattern to pop. There are different scrunching methods explained below.
   - For *smaller springy curls*, scrunch everywhere, all over your head. Flip your hair upside down and scrunch hair in the back.
   - For *smooth defined curls* from root to tips, cup a few curls at a time and scrunch with a cotton t-shirt or microfiber towel.
   - To *elongate your curls* and avoid shrinkage, use a microfiber towel to squeeze excess water and product from the middle to the ends of your hair.

4) Use a cotton t-shirt or microfiber towel to scrunch excess water and product out of your hair.
5) Air dry or diffuse hair.

Styling With Denman Brush
Using a Denman brush will give you more defined and uniform curls.

Tips for using your Denman brush:
- Only use brush on wet hair. Do not use brush on dry hair.
- Do not use brush to detangle. Detangle your hair before using a Denman brush with your fingers or a wide-tooth comb.
- Do not brush your hair without product on it.

How to style your hair with Denman Brush
1) Wash and condition hair as usual.
2) After hair is washed and completely saturated with water, apply your leave-in conditioner and cream or foam styler.
3) Taking small sections, carefully brush your hair in a downward motion.
4) After brushing each section, shake your hair to activate the curl.
5) Use a cotton t-shirt or microfiber towel to scrunch excess water and product out of your hair.
6) Air dry or diffuse hair.

Try different techniques to see what works best for you:
- For larger clumps or curls, brush downwards and flip out the ends. This technique is good for waves and looser curls.
- For medium clumps or curls, curl sections under your hair.
- For tighter, smaller, defined curls, brush hair up and away from your head.
- After you brush your hair to achieve desired look, check for fly-aways. If you find some, brush and

group them with a curls clump.

Transitioning Hair

If you are transitioning your hair and it has not fully developed its natural curl pattern yet, there are a few options. Use one of these methods to set your hair while wet:

- *Cornrows* is a hairstyle where the hair is braided very close to the scalp, using an underhand, upward motion to make a continuous, raised row.
- *Braids* is a hairstyle formed by interlacing three or more strands of hair.
- *Bantu Knots* is a hairstyle with small, coiled buns secured against the side of the head.
- *Flexi Rods* can be used to curl your hair without risking heat damage from hot tools. These bendable rods come in different sizes that you can select based on the size you want your curls.
- *Flat Twists* is a hairstyle that consists of parting the hair into cornrowed sections but flat twisting the hair and allowing them to set before unraveling them for your desired style

Once hair is completely dry, take out your hair, separate clumps and or curls, and style as desired.

CHAPTER 14
Drying and Diffusing

Once you have styled your hair as desired when wet, the next step is drying it. There are a few options when it comes to drying.

Airdry
Letting hair dry naturally requires no heat but takes longer, typically 6 or more hours. If you want maximum hair health, airdrying is best. You just have to set aside time to let your hair do what it needs to do.

Sit under a dryer
This method involves sitting under a hooded dryer. For best results, use medium to low heat. Using anything higher can unintentionally fry the hair, and we definitely don't want that to happen. Sitting under a dryer can take anywhere from 30 minutes to 2 hours, depending on your hair type and how it's styled.

Diffusing
This method involves using a handheld blow dryer with a diffuser attachment. Here is how to dry your hair using a diffuser.

1) Set your blow dryer to medium, low, or no heat. This helps reduce frizz. If you have the time, try no heat, but if you need to dry and go, aim for low heat. Under no circumstances should you go above medium heat. If the blow dryer gets too hot, don't be scared to use the cool shot setting on your blow dryer. If you don't have a low, medium, high setting on your blow dryer, then invest in a new one. You'd rather spend a couple of extra dollars on a quality hair tool than damage your hair trying to be too frugal.

2) Start with the roots. You want to focus on drying your roots first before drying the ends of your hair. They will take the longest, and your roots are the strongest.

3) Once your roots are dry, focus on the ends of your hair.

Diffusing Tips

- Once you start diffusing your hair, hands off! Unless using them to cup your hair while drying, keep your hands away from your tresses. Be sure not to disturb your curls until your hair is completely dry or else you'll cause frizz.

- Flip your head to the side to help roots and ends dry faster.

- Flip your hair upside down for added volume when diffusing your hair.

- *Once your hair is completely dry*, then you can proceed to pick out your curls and style hair as desired. You may want to use butter cream to moisturize curls, or holding spray to hold them in place.

- Drying time varies depending on the blow dryer and thickness of your hair.

- Take your time and don't rush. Beautiful curls take time and patience.

Plopping

Plopping is another method that can be used to assist in drying your hair. This involves setting your hair as usual and using a cotton t-shirt to secure your hair overnight while you sleep. This method may cause some shrinkage but will cut your drying time down significantly.

CHAPTER 15

DIY Home Recipes

Hair products can get pretty costly and expensive at times. No need to try and break the bank and purchase "the best" or most expensive products. There are several recipes you can make and cocktail up from the comfort of your own home. A lot of these ingredients you may already have in the kitchen. If not, you can find them at your local grocery store. Here are 10 recipes to get you started.

Rinse Recipes to Cleanse the Hair

Apple Cider Vinegar Rinse
Ingredients:
2 Cups of Water
¼ Cup of Apple Cider Vinegar

Directions: Combine ingredients in a bowl or applicator bottle. Wet hair, pouring mixture over hair, then scrubbing to remove build-up. The rinse can also be used after your final step of washing and conditioning your hair to help smooth cuticles and restore pH balance.

Benefits: This rinse is used to remove product build-up, restore pH balance to hair and scalp, promote blood stimulation, and encourage hair growth.

Baking Soda Rinse
2 Cups of Warm Water
½ Cup of Baking Soda

Directions: Dissolve baking soda in the warm water in an applicator bottle. Massage into hair and scalp. Consistency should be smooth and easy to apply. This mixture can be used after shampooing or in place of shampooing.

Benefits: Using this rinse leaves your hair clean, shiny, and soft. This rinse helps remove any build-up of oils, soaps, and other ingredients in typical hair care products.

Herbal Hair Rinses can be blended to achieve a specific result.

Pick the ingredients that you need for your hair:

Chamomile: Stimulates hair growth, softens hair, soothes scalp
Lavender: Stimulates hair growth
Nettle: Conditions and improves texture and/or irritated and dry scalp; helps with dandruff
Parsley: Enriches hair color and gives luster
Rosemary: Acts as a conditioner, stimulates hair growth, gives luster and body, helps with dandruff
Sage: Helps restore color to graying hair
Thyme: Good for oily hair and dandruff
Witch Hazel: Cleanses hair

Directions: After picking the ingredients that meet your hair needs, combine herbs and place in a bowl. Bring 2 cups of water to a boil, then pour herbal mixture in boiling water. Cover for 10-20 minutes, then strain mixture and allow to cool. After shampooing and conditioning, pour rinse over your hair. Leave in hair and style as usual.

Benefits: Herbal hair rinses provide deep cleansing, enrich natural hair color, soothe irritation, prevent dandruff, and stimulate the scalp to increase growth.

Deep Conditioning Recipes

Curl Defining Leave-In
Ingredients:
8 oz of your choice of conditioner with a light

consistency
5 oz Distilled Water
3 oz Aloe Vera Juice
1-2 oz Coconut Oil

Directions: Once you gather your materials in the application bottle; apply to hair while damp.

Benefits: This recipe provides moisture, definition, and shine.

Eggs and Olive Oil Recipe
Ingredients:
1 Egg Yolk
1 Tbsp of Olive Oil

Directions: Mix ingredients together in bowl. Apply mixture to hair. Let sit for 20-30 minutes. Rinse with cool or lukewarm water.

Benefits: This recipe adds protein to your hair while providing nourishment to dry or damaged hair. Please note that this recipe is enough for short or shoulder-length hair. For longer hair, add to the mixture (one egg yolk to one tbsp of olive oil).

Avocado and Mayo Recipe
Ingredients:
½ Avocado
¼ Cup Mayonnaise
2 Tbsp of Avocado Oil

Directions: Mix ingredients together in bowl. Apply mixture to hair. Let sit for 15-20 minutes. Rinse with cool or lukewarm water

Benefits: This rinse provides moisture to dry hair.

Aloe Vera Gel and Coconut Oil Recipe

Ingredients:

¼ Cup Aloe Vera Gel
2 Tbsp Coconut Oil

Directions: Mix ingredients together in bowl. Apply mixture to hair and let sit for 15 – 20 minutes. Rinse with cool or lukewarm water.

Benefits: This recipe promotes hair growth, adds moisture, and helps with dandruff in your hair.

Greek Yogurt, Apple Cider, and Honey
Ingredients:
½ Cup of Greek Yogurt
1 Tbsp Apple Cider Vinegar
1 Tbsp Honey
Lavender Oil

Directions: Mix ingredients together in bowl. Apply mixture to hair and let sit for 15 – 20 minutes. Rinse with cool or lukewarm water

Benefits: Every ingredient in this mixture serves a distinct purpose. Yogurt adds protein to your hair, and apple cider helps cleanse and detangle. Honey locks in moisture. Lavender oil helps mask the smell.

Hair Mask Recipes

Honey, Egg, Apple Cider Vinegar Mask
Ingredients:
1 Teaspoon Honey
1 Egg
1 Tbsp Apple Cider Vinegar

Directions: Combine ingredients in a small bowl. The recipe can be doubled depending on the length of your hair. Leave mask on hair for 30-40 minutes before rinsing. Recipe is nourishing for ALL hair types.

Benefits: This recipe is a hydrating recipe that provides shine and nourishes hair without weighing it down.

Coconut Oil, Sugar, and Essential Oil Mask
Ingredients:
2 Tbsp Raw Unrefined Coconut Oil
4 Teaspoons Raw Sugar
5 Drops Peppermint Oil
2 Drops Tea Tree Oil

Directions: Mix ingredients together in a small bowl. Using your fingertips or a color application brush, apply mixture directly in 2-inch sections to clean damp hair while in the shower. Once mixture is applied evenly, massage hair for 1-3 minutes, clip your hair up, and leave in hair for the duration of your shower. Rinse hair before getting out of shower and style hair as usual.

Benefits: This treatment helps remove and reduce flakes caused by dandruff.

I hope at least one of these DIY recipes can save you a little money and help you on your natural hair journey!

CHAPTER 16
Protective Styles

Transitioning to natural hair can be a process in itself. You may not be all for the "Big Chop," and that's completely fine. Here are a few protective hairstyles that can help you on your journey while letting your hair grow out. There are several benefits to wearing protective hairstyles: they protect your hair from harsh outside elements, help maintain moisture in your hair, assist with length retention, and of course, are stylish. Everyone's hair and hairstyles are different; it's just a matter of finding out which one you like best and what works for you. Here are 10 protective styles to get you started.

Examples of Protective Styles:

Braids – There are so many different styles to choose from. Braids are low maintenance and can last for weeks. Section hair to the braid size you prefer. Divide that section into three equal sections, then braid down as you would traditionally braid your hair.

Flat Twist – Similar to cornrows, flat twists have the same effect but are lighter and easier to wear.

Two Strand Twist – Individual twists add texture to your hair and are easy to maintain. Divide hair into sections and twist hair like usual. The difference is that this time, like cornrows, you'll add strands as you twist down your hair to the nape of your neck. Once you reach the bottom of your scalp, twist hair into two-strand twists.

Buns – There are several types of buns you can wear from messy buns, doughnut buns, ninja buns, and more. They are a good go-to for something quick when you are pressed for time and on the go. Use gel to slick hair into a high, mid, or low ponytail, then wrap hair into a bun.

Space Buns – This is a fun protective style. Divide your hair down the middle and place a high bun on the top of your head to get the look.

Cornrows – Cornrows are a popular and classic braided hairstyle that requires little maintenance. Hair can be added for length and to make them last longer. Section hair starting at the front from the root, then split that section into three sections. Braid hair as you normally would but grab a small section of hair as you braid down to the back of your head. Once you reach the bottom of your scalp, continue to braid hair as usual. Secure the bottom of the hair with the elastic.

Bantu Knots – This was a popular style in the '90s, but is making a comeback. Section hair and twist from root to ends until hair starts to twist into itself. Form twist into a bun on the top of your hair and secure small bun into place.

Halo Braid – A popular up style hairdo, halo braids keeps hair out of your face and still protects your hair. Gather all of your hair into one braid and wrap hair around your head like a "halo."

Crochet Braids – This style takes less time than individuals but still give the braids look. Braid your hair into cornrows, then crochet braids into hair under cornrows.

Two Strand Twists – This is a quick and easy way to style your hair. Taking small sections of hair, twist strands in opposite directions, then twist together to create two-strand twists. Twist hair for roots to the ends to complete the look.

Finger Waves- This is a hairstyle that was popular in the '20s,

'30s, and '90s, and has made a comeback again. This style involves applying gel to hair and creating an "S" shape similar to a wave with your finger, hence the name "finger wave."

CHAPTER 17
Heat Damage

While we are on our natural hair journey, we need to realize and accept that heat is NOT our friend. Heat damage is caused by too much heat being applied to your hair. Heat damage can cause your hair to lie flat, release natural curls, release moisture, and hold a different shape than your hair would have if the heat wasn't applied. It can also dry out the cuticle of your hair and cause the structure to change.

Once you experience hair damage, sometimes you may feel like the only way to revive it is to do the "Big Chop." Some of us are not that bold. If you're not ready to cut all the damaged hair at one time or you want to transition your locks, depending on the amount of heat damage, there are a few things you can do to revive your locks.

Tips for reviving heat damaged hair:

- Wear protective hairstyles while your hair transitions.
- Try finger combing hair instead of using detangling combs and brushes.
- Deep condition hair weekly.
- Use hair masks and/or hair treatments to assist in reviving your locks.
- Maintain a good moisture routine for your hair moisturizers as explained in detail in Chapter 9. Be sure to keep your ends moisturized because they tend to be the driest.
- Moisturize as often as your hair requires it daily, every other day, or weekly.

-    Try to use the least amount of heat as possible when styling your hair; the less heat, the better.
-    If you do use heat, try to preserve your hair by wrapping it or pin curling it at night.
- If you do experience heat damage, be patient and understand it will take some time for your hair to become healthy again.
-    If your hair is damaged beyond repair, really consider the big chop and wearing protective styles. Alternatively, you can trim your hair a little at a time. Whatever you decide, I'm sure you will love your real natural locks without any heat or chemicals.

CHAPTER 18
How to Sleep with Curls Overnight

Once you get your curls, another challenge you may be faced with is making them last. Of course, that includes how to sleep with them and make them last overnight. Everybody's hair is different, but here are a few techniques you can try. It's just a matter of finding out what works best for you. If done correctly, curls can last at least a week, if not longer,

One thing all of these methods have in common is silk. Whether it be a silk scarf, silk bonnet, or a silk pillowcase, using silk materials will help preserve your curls and prevent breakage. All of these methods are demonstrated in the YouTube video, you can find by following the link below.
https://youtu.be/E9lFxL627-o

Method 1
Sleep on a Satin Pillowcase - Some choose not to do anything but use a silk pillowcase while sleeping to preserve curls. This is a great option for those who just want to go to sleep each night without worrying about their tresses.

Method 2
Pineapple - This method includes gathering your hair to the top of your head and securing loosely with an elastic band. Afterward you can secure with a silk scarf or sleep on a silk pillowcase.

Method 3
Upside Down Scarf Method - This method involves flipping your

hair upside down and securing your hair with a silk scarf, where all of your hair is gathered at the top of your head. Once you secure with a silk scarf, the curls will be falling out of the top of the scarf. At this point all you need to do is tuck your curls into the top, then secure the top part of your scarf by twisting and tucking that in as well. This method is personally one of my favorites.

Method 4
Silk Scarf and Bonnet Method – This method is very similar to the Upside-Down Scarf Method. It involves flipping your hair upside down and securing your hair with a silk scarf, leaving all of your curls gathered at the top of your hair. Instead of tucking your curls and tucking your silk scarf, you would put a silk bonnet over the loose curls at the top of your head.

Method 5
Silk Bonnet Method - This method involves securing your hair with a silk bonnet. Just place the bonnet on your head and tuck your curls in.

These are a few methods to get you started. I hope one of these methods works well for you.

CHAPTER 19
Helpful Hair Tips for Your Natural Hair Journey

- Choose hair products wisely. Always make sure to read the ingredients, so you know what you are putting in your hair.
- Lay off the heat as much as you can. Remember, heat is NOT your friend!
- When detangling, section your hair to make it easier and reduce breakage.
- Keep in mind chemicals, such as relaxers, perms, hair dye, and texturizers can also damage hair, causing it to break. Be mindful when using these products.
- Sleep with a silk scarf, bonnet, or pillowcase. This will minimize the damage done to your hair.
- Trim ends regularly. Depending on how fast your hair grows, every 2-3 months is a good start.
- Develop a healthy hair routine that includes shampooing, conditioning, deep conditioning, treatments, and masks. (Masks are optional depending on the condition of your hair)
- Deep condition regularly. Whether you choose to use masks and treatments is optional, but deep conditioning should definitely be a part of your routine.
- Scalp massages help with the blood flow circulation to your scalp and are also a good way to assist in hair growth.
- Use cool or cold water when washing hair. This will close the cuticle and help retain moisture.
- Taking hair vitamins can assist in growing your hair strong and healthy.
- Comb your hair starting from the ends and work your way up

to the roots. This will help prevent breakage.
- Use product "cocktailing" to moisturize and hydrate hair.
-   Use a diffuser when drying hair to even out your curl pattern and add body.
-   Use elastic bands to secure hair instead of rubber bands to reduce breakage.
-   Remember transitioning to natural hair does not happen overnight. Take your time, be patient, and don't get frustrated. Learn to love your tresses.

These are just a few tips to help you on your natural hair journey. So, there you have a step by step guide to achieving and transitioning to natural hair. I hope you enjoyed this manual and find this information useful to you on your natural hair journey. I hope it helps you reach your natural hair goals in no time!

CHAPTER 20
Definition of Terms

Clarifying Shampoo – shampoos that are designed to remove surface-level gunk and grime, rather than condition and smooth; deep cleanses your hair from chemicals, waxes, and residue left behind by your hair products

Co-Wash – using conditioner in the place of shampoo

Coily Hair – Type 4 hair, the tightest among all hair types; curls spring straight from scalp

Curl Activator – product used to provide moisture to fight frizz and promote shine; helps define curls.

Curl Cream – product designed to moisturize, smooth, and define your curls; aids in providing soft hold and definition to your curls

Curl Smoothies – hair product whose primary function is to soften, moisturize, refresh, detangle, condition, and style hair

Curly Hair - hair that is a spiral shape; ranges from loose to tight

Deep Condition – hair product whose purpose is to provide intense conditioning to the hair

Denman Brush – hairbrush designed to give you more defined and uniformed curls

Density – refers to the number of hair strands on your head; it is determined by how close your strands are to each other and describes how thin or thick your hair appears

Detangle – removing tangle from hair

Diffusing – hair drying method that involves using a handheld blow dryer with a diffuser attachment.

Gels - hair styling product use to harden hair into a particular hairstyle

Hair Milk – hydrating leave-in that aids in detangling and combating frizz

Hair pattern - identified by the shape of the hair strands; ranges from kinky, curvy, or winding around themselves into spirals

Heat Damage – damage done to your hair as a result of too much heat being applied

Kinky Hair – Type 4a-4c hair that is tightly coiled with a zig-zag pattern

Masks - a deep conditioning treatment that helps heal damaged hair

Moisturizer – hair product whose purpose is to add moisture to your hair

Mousse – hair product used for reviving curl definition and fighting frizz

Natural Hair - hair that has not been "altered" or processed by any type of chemical, including straighteners, relaxers, and texturizers.

Plopping – hair drying method involves setting your hair and using a cotton t-shirt to secure hair overnight while you sleep

Pomades – hair product used for hold, shine, and controlling frizz; locks in moisture and often contains wax to help with hold

Porosity – hair's ability to absorb and retain moisture

Protective Hairstyle - any style that keeps the ends of the hair tucked away and minimizes manipulation

Pre-poo - process of applying treatment to the hair before the shampooing; purpose of this treatment is to provide your hair with a protective layer

Reconstructor – hair product used to make the hair stronger; generally protein-based

Relaxer - lotion or cream that makes the hair easier to straighten and manage

Rinse – using water to remove or wash out product from hair

Scrubs – hair product whose purpose is purifying the scalp for bright and healthy hair

Sealant - helps to seal in moisture and provides moisturizing properties; penetrates the hair shaft with the help of water

Shampoo – liquid haircare cleansing product used for cleaning hair

Shrinkage - decrease in length when your hair dries

Straight Hair - Type 1 Hair that develops its structure from the shape of the cortex; fibers of the hair are round, making it drop evenly on all sides of the scalp

Straighteners - is a hair styling technique involving the flattening and straightening of hair in order to give it a smooth, streamlined, and sleek appearance

Strand Size - the width, thickness, or circumference of the individual hair strands

Texturizers – a chemical process that smooths and de-frizzes your hair while maintaining some of your natural curls

Transitioning – the period it takes to get the chemicals out of your hair

Treatments – penetrates the hair, restoring and maintaining internal strength; 2 types of treatments are reconstructors and moisturizers.

Wavy Hair - Type 2 hair that has a slight bump and a visible S pattern

Index